The Origin of Your Health:

A 4-week course in realizing your optimal wellness

By Rob Wright C.P.T.

Many know this story… The time comes when we wish to take control of our wellness. Either a look in the mirror, a new struggle with an old pair of pants that used to slide on with ease, a doctor's suggestion that it is time to exercise and change eating habits or risk further disease, or a desire to run a 5k for a good cause brings us into yet another gym with more peppy trainers, more confusing equipment, more feelings of judgement, more opportunities for self-sabotage, and more presumed disappointment.

We have seen our spouse, friend, or coworker have great success in changing their health and fitness, but we have failed before, or have hit a frustrating plateau. Why will it be different this time?

Why does it seem easy for others but not for me?

Am I unlucky? Doomed by genetics? Too lazy? Unmotivated? Too unhealthy? Too busy? Hate exercise and diet?

This 4-week program will assist you in realizing the origin of your health and wellness. Included are reading materials and exercises to help you overcome unhealthy paradigms that lead to a sense of powerlessness over your own wellbeing. Over the next four weeks, you will become more present with your physical being. This program will also allow you to quiet the mind and understand subconscious programming that can contribute to creating disease and disorder within the body.

Realizing these subconscious patterns can:

- Improve self-motivation
- Help you identify unhealthy programming
- Reestablish a healthy body image
- Allow you to love your body now, even though you wish to make healthy improvements
- Show you why you may have been unsuccessful in reclaiming your health in the past with diets and exercise.

The greatest thing you can do to improve your health is to know yourself fully. We could spend years identifying all of the negative things in the world that could affect your health from foods to pathogens to lifestyles, but in the end, the key is in knowing yourself. With simple mindfulness techniques, you will start to see these patterns of thought and action that keep you from realizing perfect health and wellness. When we can see these untruths that creep into our subconscious, we will find it effortless to set a goal and achieve it, even though it seemed to be an uphill battle before.

Dive into these exercises and be completely honest with yourself. This is not the time to push aside negative thoughts or emotions. Instead, it is the time to face them head on, feel them, and bring light into the darkness. I wish you luck and blessings on this journey to the center of your being. This is where healing happens. This is where optimal health is realized. At this center, you will reprogram every cell in your body to work in concert with your mind and spirit.

In less than one year, 98% of the cells in your body are brand new! The other 2% (collagen and connective tissue) take just over a year to replenish. Therefore, in just over a year, you can rebuild your entire body, cell-by-cell.

This is incredible news. This shows that you, *the real you*, are NOT your body. There is not one, single cell that has been with you since birth. The physical state you currently see in the mirror and take to the doctor have been built by your nutrition, activity, mental and emotional state, and other external factors including toxins in the air, food, and water. Your body is a reflection of your life in totality.

The good news is, you can choose, at great extent, to what your body is subjected. (Food, exercise, plenty of water, proper breathing, etc.) And the things we cannot immediately control (toxins, stress, etc.), we can limit their impact with techniques and appropriate cleansing.

Stress has a huge impact on our body. The following are just some of the effects:

- Headaches
- High blood pressure
- Digestive issues
- Lower immune system
- Sleeping problems

"Any condition caused or worsened by stress can be alleviated through meditation"

"Relaxation response helps metabolism, lowers blood pressure, improves heart rate, breathing, and brainwaves."

—Cardiologist, Dr. Herbert Benson MD

With this information, I challenge you to rebuild your entire body over the next year, cell by cell, with care and purpose. This is how you can reclaim your health. This is how you can honor your body and, in turn, yourself. It is not necessary to experience more frustration and disappointment, for…

"Natural forces within us are the true healers of disease."

—Hippocrates

Week 1

'Defining' Your Body

What is your body? Is it a cluster of cells, playing roles as needed forming muscles, bones, tendons, teeth, nails, hair, organs, and eyeballs? Or is it just this cumbersome thing your mind drags around daily, frustratingly lagging behind the sprinting gray matter ahead. Could it be your instrument with the perfectly polished brass of a beckoning trumpet, or elegantly finished baby grand piano that need not even be played to display its beauty? Is it your hammer and nail, as an athlete or physical laborer? Maybe it houses a mind that crunches numbers, builds bridges, or ponders the imponderable. We know this much, it is yours. How you view it, use it, and for what end and purpose is completely up to you, and if it is running at its highest potential, your path becomes easier to navigate.

What is your body for? Now, this question could be answered as pragmatically or existentially as you wish, but it should be answered in some fashion. What does it do for me? What does it symbolize, and what is it truly? To determine the best workout regimen for you, figure out the needs you are and are not currently meeting for your particular body and the way you use it to experience your unique life. Factor in your body type, current strengths, weaknesses, and imbalances and you have a great start to thoroughly examining your approach to training. This applies to beginners as well as seasoned "fitness-enthusiasts".

Some of us have spent year by year, sweating and grunting in the gym… and sweating and grunting at home as we slide our chair up to a table that displays a strict, clean meal that resembles nothing like the pizza we are craving. It is easy to fall into routine, hit a plateau, or just jump in to the newest fad training or nutritional program that rears its head. Always reevaluate yourself and where your fitness program entwines with you and your bodily changes over time with new or different needs.

Most of us, when we pause to examine the existential and philosophical angle of the physical being, conclude we should view our body as very important, even sacred. It is our link to the earth and vessel for our soul. Therefore, it obviously should be treated with respect and care—Yes, for the amazing instrument that it is, but also so there can be as little inhibition as possible, while serving as your tool and your home throughout whatever your adventure is and shall be. Your body serves you—for life. Treat it as such. Your body is the very tip of the arrow with which you pierce this world and experience your life story. It is your defense and your haven. The body forges ahead, through the sometimes hazardous maze of life. If it is in balance, the hazards become less, your spirit will breathe easier, and your mind will be sharper and better attuned than before.

What is your body telling you? Take time to assess your entire physical being. Examine every cell with intention. Listen closely for its response. A slight ache here… a buzzing there…

slight muscle twitch here or there... swelling... itching... cramping... emanating heat or cold... on and on and on. Any little thing could be a message. Feel it and take notice. The more you become in tune with the subtle signs your body expresses, the easier it will be to prevent and avoid sickness and correct imbalance. Be fully present with your body!

I understand that some could take this too far... Do not examine simply looking for things that are wrong. I really don't want to encourage hypochondria. There will be many areas of your body that will feel spot on. Take note of muscle groups that feel relaxed, yet strong. In what areas are your best bone alignments, skin, flexibility and strengths? How have you treated those areas as opposed to the ones that are imbalanced? What steps would it take to begin aligning and nourishing your body properly? Each person reading will have definite, unique needs when addressing their program or nutrition. Know your body first; it will be a tremendous help when determining where and if to search for professional services or advice. Listen to that body. It will alert you of some impressive things, and even teach you how to care for it properly. The body speaks to us every day, from sun up to sun down.

After truly knowing what your body is, does, and says, you will find physical balance and a healthy, while extremely manageable, lifestyle. If you fight it and make it a struggle or conjure fictitious ways in which your body is insufficient for you, those old, tough junkyard dogs of new diets and more gym hours will be chomping at your heels, only leading to frustration and minimal success. Once you see your physical self for what it is to you, and why it is the way it is right now, your health pursuit will then become effortless.

Exercises:

Meditations:

Sit silently and focus on the following questions. Take notes of your answers and realizations throughout this course.

1. How do you view your body?

2. What is the body? What does it mean to you both philosophically and practically?

3. What is your body's potential?

Mindfulness exercises (Being aware, observing during active life):

Throughout the week, observe without judgment, your body's functions. Be present with every ache and pain. Be aware of what feels good and strong within your body as well. Notice the tiniest details including times of cravings, nervous mannerisms, and the thoughts that coincide with these.

- Notice the thoughts and emotions that come up while preparing your meals, during meals, and after meals.

- How does your body feel after eating different foods or consuming other substances? Compare and contrast.

- How does your body feel before and after exercise? How does it feel on a day with or without exercise? How does this correlate with mood, thoughts, cravings, aches and pains, etc?

Weekly quote:

**"Be careful when reading health books,
you may die of a misprint."**

—Mark Twain

Sometimes, we just need to laugh.

This week has been about observing your body and how the mind reacts throughout your day. You are getting to know your physical being.

Week 2

Optimal Health and its Origin

Health—One of, if not the main issue concerning our society is swimming in our heads from sun up to sun down, and we find ourselves chasing the proverbial wild goose trying to discern which path to take to unlock our healthiest self. There is no study needed, no experiment necessary to prove, that a healthier you will improve all areas of your life, mentally, creatively, emotionally, and socially. We see that every day.

Where does your health come from? Modern thought mixes genetic and external factors for the bases of most procedural medicine, diagnoses, and therapy. Therefore, this creates the philosophy of dodging the things you cannot possibly control to attain optimal health. Play your cards as dealt.

Many people, including medical professionals, are continually awakening to the obvious defect in that philosophy. Science clearly shows the effects of stress and poor diet. This is obviously a major area that *can* be controlled. So why are many people, when shown the benefits of happiness and good nutrition, choosing to be unhealthy? Yes… I said choosing.

Where does the line end, though? At what point do our *choices* and our predetermined *"luck"* fork in the journey? Or does it?

The philosophy to which many are turning new eyes is a philosophy of many ancient cultures, and much of these are still practiced today all over the world, and now starting to boom in America. Ironically, the Native Americans practiced much of this, so it is hardly a new concept to our soil. These old paths are being explored again, and we have all been hearing about the necessity of mind, body, and spirit balance. If these are aligned, one can assume good health. (…and "REsume" good health as well).

I see the change ahead, and have been blessed to see it working everywhere, daily. There has been a shift in how we view our health and wellbeing. It is a change deviating from the current thinking that has proven to be ineffective and costly. The economics do not make sense; neither do the results and efficacy of some modern paths. There are a lot of new possibilities ahead, with limitless reason for optimism. We just need to find that balance.

But what are we balancing? Well, mind, body, and spirit. Are the mind, body, and soul one? Should they be treated as one? Is there a ring leader?

The body is your physical, flesh and bone stuff that maintains all the processes you need to experience life on earth. Consider it the grand machine, but do not dishonor it by thinking it only mechanical. It is very much organic and alive. Honestly the body can be the pawn in this game of life, at the mercy of the mind and the soul. At the same time, it is our temple and the very vessel that makes this incredible journey possible. Both seemingly insignificant yet indeed a keystone of life; it is the first thing most see of our being. It is what plagues or boosts us. What is it a representation of? Why is it the way that it is, and to what end or purpose? It is this: Our poor physical health is the physical manifestation of the struggle between our mind and our spirit.

The mind, oh the mind… What a grand cathedral of human evolution!! We hold it up, saying, "Look!! Look at what this blob of grey matter can do!!! Oh, how we have come so far as a species," when in fact, the brain is a computer. The brain is *not* the mind. I would put it in the same category as the body, except for a tricky little thing. The brain can be programmed by both external and internal stimuli… A computer that can program itself! This is where the mind comes in. That is, if you let it continue on, set to a certain frequency. It goes about its business, controlling all the involuntary goings-on within the various systems of the body. Usually, we are only aware of it when it acts up, bringing us to analyzing and thinking, or distracting us from a task. Sometimes thoughts of worry or pressure arise. These are all constructed by the mind, using the brain to sense and process all around it. If left unchecked, it will do its best to keep the physical body safe, but it will program the brain based on a paradigm of fear. The mind looks out only for the mind and the body can be left to fend for itself.

The brain that processes conscious negative thought also programs the involuntary actions of the physical body, right down to the cellular level. Science has found that peptides are released according to different emotional states, triggering immediate responses within EVERY cell in your body. If staying in a state of perpetual depression, your cells will be programmed thoroughly and react accordingly.

Take that a step farther... The same mind that thinks a negative thought, also controls the subconscious, and if habitual, decides the workings of the involuntary processes of the body through the wiring of the brain. One of these processes most immediately affected is the immune system.

If you continue on a negative or depressed, fearful or angry pathway of thinking, each cell grows and performs according to these signals, hormones, and peptides released by the brain. If that source is corrupted through negative emotion or thought, the molecules released for normal function of systems gets constantly mixed with those negatively thought provoked, survival triggered compounds, therefore ensuring the outcome at the cellular level to be less than optimal, at best.

Imagine a river being fed both by a beautiful, clean spring from one side, and on the other side, runoff from a toxic waste facility. Is not the whole river and whatever it feeds into poisoned? "Oh, but by the time it gets to me, it will be diluted... Only just a little bit of poison..."

Well, that little bit of poison continually feeds those recycling cells, from birth to death, day by day, month by month, on and on. This is what we are building our bodies with, using the very basic building blocks of life. They deserve the best start they can get.

So, it's virtually two on one against the spirit. The spirit, despite its current dwelling, is a free flowing embodiment of light. It is connected to pure consciousness. Despite popular belief, you are not your thoughts, or your body. As previously mentioned, 98% of the cells in your body completely regenerate in less than one year. (Collagen and cartilage take a bit longer.) Therefore, the only thing left standing that is truly you, year by year, is your consciousness—intact and never affected by any physical change. It stands to reason that the only unchanging, eternal part of you is the best place to start the reprogramming process, en route to controlling the mind and manifesting the physical health you deserve. Yes—deserve.

By connecting regularly to our spirit, which is more intimately connected with pure consciousness, we can bypass the negative reactionary mind, infusing our health with proactive choices that benefit our physical being.

Remember earlier I mentioned "choosing" poor health? At this point in society, with all the education available, it's only responsible that we come to the recognition that many people are choosing poor health. Working in the fitness and health field for the last several years, I have heard every excuse why someone cannot make a workout appointment or follow a better diet. From "I don't have the time with work and this and this…" to "My kids and husband will never eat that, and I'm not cooking two meals…" There are a million reasons in between.

Think about that for a minute…

I know we live in a busy, uncertain world. We have placed so many demands on ourselves, that there are no more minutes left even for our own basic well-being. At the end of the day, as our aches and pains grow and we complain about the unsung power of an M&M's addiction, and our pants don't fit, can't sleep, sad all day and night, anxious, nervous, itchy, flaky, watery eyes, nasal congestion, spare tire, and on and on and on… At some point, we need to look in the mirror and make new choices. Why do I not have ten extra minutes to eat a healthy breakfast? Of course, you do have time if your health is truly a priority. It's about wanting to utilize the time.

The likelihood of ten more minutes of sleep doing anything to drastically alter your day's productivity and/or happiness is silly. Here, we are choosing to skip breakfast for something practically inconsequential. It sounds silly, and it's easy to shake my personal trainer finger at you and say, "Now, now, you certainly know better," but what does that really accomplish? Nothing.

We are deliberately CHOOSING something rather insignificant over very basic needs, proven by the most basic of sciences of how our body works.

The fact is, and a slightly jarring one at first to most people is this: For whatever reason, and one that can be pinpointed only personally through inward focus, you somehow feel you are not worthy of caring for your body properly. Somewhere along your journey, your mind became programmed into thinking the trivial mattered and the important does not. How and why did this programming happen?

It all comes down to self-realization. Once you realize who you truly are, you can then take the reins, ignoring the programming of the mind's conscious negative thought, while reprogramming all of the involuntary processes that need balancing with positive thought and expression. You will see how much you truly deserve the highest possible health! Once knowing this, it will be harder to make the excuses…

This is the future: Connecting to spirit → control of conscious mind, producing healthier sub-conscious → healthier sub-conscious mind sets in rhythm the body's processes, naturally, and organically, allowing us to make better lifestyle choices.

We need to stop chasing that sick wild goose and tripping over our bandages. Go to the source of it all. Heal our spirit by owning it, recognizing it as our true being-ness, and being grateful for it. That is where our true health resides.

We had been going about it like this: Physical body shows symptom → Diagnose and treat symptom; if symptom persists or worsens, spreads to other areas, etc. → we *might* trace it to the mind → once we get to the mind, we end there. Good luck.

As we start to observe our thoughts and set new patterns of positive thinking, so will be the same process of each cell in your body. Imagine practicing this for an entire year… Every cell of your body will have been placed by a bricklayer who cared so deeply for their home, that nothing could invade or disrupt its bliss. That is optimal health.

Exercises:

Meditations: (Contemplate these questions)

1. What are your biggest stressors?

2. When were you first noticing disease, unhealthiness, or imbalance in your physical being? What was occurring in your life at the time of this? What lead up to this moment?

3. When was the last time you felt you were in the best shape of your life or at your optimal health? What was happening in your life at this time?

4. What are some untruths about health that you have previously held as truths?

5. If you were to rebuild your body, cell by cell, what would it look like, feel like, and what would you do with it that you cannot do presently? What is optimal health to YOU?

Mindfulness exercises:

- This week, spend time observing the mind, reflecting on life and how your mind reacts to memories, relationships, and how this might affect your wellness.

- Is your mind calm? Is it disruptive? Are you in control of it, or is does it control you and your daily routines?

- What are your fears? What do you find yourself worrying about? What can you control? What is out of your control?

- What quiets your mind and puts your body at ease? What motivates you to do the work to improve your health? What mental actions demotivate you?

Weekly Quote:

"Surgeons can cut out anything except cause."

—Herbert M. Shelton

Week 3

Dr. Masaru Emoto conducted an experiment showing that specific blessings affected the molecular structure of water. In this experiment, monks blessed water before it was frozen. Each blessing showed a different outcome in the water crystals that appeared.

The study went as far as showing the difference between polluted water, before and after. With a blessing, even polluted water can become drinkale through only positive thought! This study should open some eyes about the potential of intention.

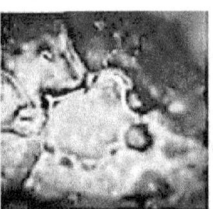
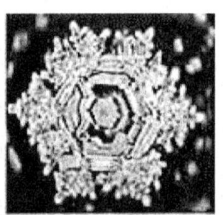

Water Molecule,
Before Offering a Prayer

Water Molecule,
After Offering a Prayer

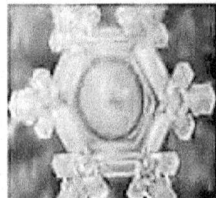
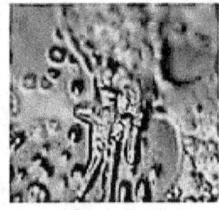
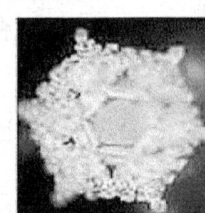

Thank You

You Make Me Sick,
I Will Kill You

Love and Apprecia

Our bodies are approximately 65% water, varying due to age, gender, health, and weight. Knowing this and seeing the effect of the water blessing experiment, our conscious thought and other intentional stimuli can greatly affect our wellbeing. If you think illness, illness will come or continue. If you imbue your body, mind, and spirit with health affirming, loving, grateful, thoughts and stimuli, your body will respond positively. This is the key in rebuilding your body, cell by cell. About 2/3 of our body's water is within the cells themselves—bones, skin, organs, everything.

The food we eat also contains a large amount of water. The quality of the water we drink is incredibly important. Being present with this will truly make a difference in our health.

Meditations:

1. Sit in silence sending love and appreciation to every cell in your body. Visualize your cells becoming healthier. Become aware of how your body feels before and after this meditation.

2. What negative stimuli have you been sending your body? What changes can be made?

Mindfulness exercises:

- Prepare each meal with love and appreciation. Ask your body to be open to receive each meal for fuel, rebuilding, and nourishment.

- Bless the water you drink and the food you eat.

- Thank your body for its functions and the tasks you require from it.

Weekly quote:

"Every human being is the author of
his own health or disease."
—Guatama Buddha

Week 4

Realizing Your Perfect Health

When we wish for something to change or improve, we find ourselves focusing on what is wrong. Though it is important to see where the problem lies, dwelling on the problem does not make it disappear. Our body is the expression of the past and present state of our mental doings and physical actions. All of our experiences and our perceptions of them become manifest as the dwelling for our spirit.

Yes, we want improved health. We wish to be free of disease and age more slowly. We want to look better, feel better, and do better. However, this attachment to controlled change can bury the beauty and perfection of our current state of being. The biggest secret for optimal health is realizing your present perfection. The presence of disease or undesired health does not mean that you are flawed in any way. These manifestations are lessons. Just as every scar has a story, each physiological symptom of dis-ease has an origin and a backstory. Our experiences shape us and forge strength, wisdom, and faith. Your health, as it is NOW, is perfect, and right as it needs to be for your current state of living.

Your current state of physical being will change no matter what is done. From this point of "now" is where you can determine how it changes by the choices you make and the perception you have of your wellness and state of being. You are not the body, but the body is an aspect of you. You are the chooser. You can choose how you view your nutrition, your activities, and what limitations you place on them. No matter how you look, feel, or think right now, there is always a positive way forward. Change will happen. What the results of change are will depend on the force that causes the change. You are that force, both in the subtle ways and the palpable ways. No matter how unhealthy the body may be, there is always something that you can do to alter the course of change for the better.

Exercises:

Meditations:

1. What do you feel you cannot overcome? Is it truth or untruth?

2. Why does life interfere with your health? How does your health interfere with life?

3. What immediate changes do you need to make to manifest your optimal health?

Recharging meditation to open up and heal every cell in the body:

Try to do this during daylight time, utilizing the transformational energy and life giving power of the sun. Perform this meditation at least once and whenever needed to recharge if you have found it enjoyable and effective.

Focus on deep breathing, inhaling new breath at a count of 4 seconds, exhaling old for 6 seconds

Become fully present with your body. Start at the top of your head. Visualize every cell opening up and filled with golden light. Each body part will be a cluster of millions of tiny sun-like cells.

For the head, for example, start with the brain, then scalp, eyes, nose, bones, ears, mouth, teeth, etc. Try to visualize each and every part of your physical makeup. Continue this throughout body. Include organs, connective tissue, skin, muscles, blood cells, etcetera until your entire body is comprised of fresh, sun-like golden cells.

Feel your body. Take notice of what feels great and what feels off. Bring your awareness to what feels off and spend more time in that area, visualizing the cells opening, blood flow going to and from, and golden light. See what thoughts, images, and messages come with focusing on those areas.

Finally, see your body as it is now. Visualize a fire and step into it. As you step out of the fire, see your new body as you conceptualize perfect health. Interact with the "new" you. Ask your healthy physical being what it took for this to occur.

Weekly quote:

"The art of medicine consists of amusing the patient while nature cures the disease."
—Voltaire

Thank you for taking this journey. I hope that this has helped you come to realizations about your perception of health and where it originates. If there are any questions, feel free to send an email. If you are looking for further guidance with exercise and/or nutrition, I do offer customized programs that can accommodate any state of health or level of fitness. Simply inquire about these programs, and I will be happy to provide more information.

Blessings,

Rob Wright
wright.training101@gmail.com